Cure Sore Throats, Colds and Coughs with Cayenne Pepper

NIGEL THOMAS

ISBN – 13: 978-1482380958
ISBN – 10: 1482380951

Cover Photo Acknowledgement
Paul from FreedigitalPhotos.net

DEDICATION

This book is dedicated to all those who seek an alternative way of treating their health issues.

I wish you all a long and healthy life.

CONTENTS

ACKNOWLEDGMENTS

I would like to acknowledge all the help and encouragement my wife Jane has given me in the writing of this book. I would also like to thank my daughter Claire for her support too.

Without these two in my life this book would probably have never been written.

INTRODUCTION

Around the world people spend a fortune each year trying to eliminate the symptoms of a common cold.

At the first sign of their symptoms they start buying highly priced remedies whose only benefit seems to for the big drug companies themselves.

What this book aims to show is that there is a real natural alternative to over the counter products, that is not only better but, more importantly, costs a fraction of the price too.

The common cold is something that all of us have suffered with from time to time, some more often than others. For some the effects are far worse than for other people.

But the symptoms remain the same for all of us, a

sore throat and blocked nose, followed by sneezing leading to a runny nose and eventually ending with a cough. All in all you simply feel down-right unwell.

These symptoms usually feel worse during the first two or three days and particularly at night time. Normally a cold will last for about a week, although the after effects of the cough can make it last longer.

The best advice for anyone suffering from a common cold is to stay at home, keep warm, drink plenty of fluids and rest up until the symptoms have passed.

In fact it's estimated that in the USA alone more than twenty-two million school days are lost each year due to the common cold.

But, let's be honest, few of us can really stay at home each time we get a cold, especially as the average adult suffers around two colds a year.

The majority of us have jobs to keep, busy lives to lead and, if taking time off work means losing money, bills to pay too. It is just not feasible to let the symptoms of a cold rule our lives.

So how do we catch the common cold?

The common cold is a virus that is passed from one person to another. If, for example, someone with the cold virus covers their mouth with their hand while coughing, then uses the same hand to touch a door handle, the next person to touch that handle stands a pretty good chance of catching the virus too.

The closer we are to people the easier it is to pass the virus around, especially among family members and work colleagues.

What is needed is a product readily at hand that can be taken as soon as we feel a cold coming on that will rapidly get to work to relieve the symptoms and cure the cold as quickly as possible.

A NATURAL CURE FOR SORE THROATS, COLDS AND COUGHS

The usual approach to curing the common cold, or at least coping with it, is to visit your local pharmacist or drug store and buy an array of different products all claiming to be the miracle cure.

These products range from throat lozenges for your sore throat. Menthol sweets that help you breathe more easily. Paracetamol tablets that help dry up your runny nose. And tonics that help you sleep more easily at night.

And that doesn't include the whole range of different cough mixtures that ease your ticklish cough, your dry cough or your chesty cough.

The big drug companies (see Drug Companies) have certainly latched onto a money maker here.

But instead of paying good hard earned money for all those different over the counter products, why not try an alternative?

This product cannot only alleviate most, or all, of the symptoms but is natural and free from additives too.

You won't find this particular product on a drug store shelf though. You will, more probably, find it in your local health food shop or maybe even at the back of your kitchen cupboard.

Because the natural product we are talking about is cayenne pepper!

And this really does have the right to be called a miracle cure.

So what's so good about cayenne pepper?

For hundreds of years cayenne pepper, or Capsicum as it is sometimes also known, has been used as not only a flavoring for meals but also for its many different health benefits. These health benefits are far to numerous to mention here (see Benefits at a Glance) but trust me when I say they range from the digestive system, the heart and blood vessels, the prostate, and many other major organs too.

In fact cayenne pepper is well known for fortifying the overall health of your entire body.

And the good news for us is that it is also a fantastic cure for the symptoms of a common cold too.

HOW TO USE CAYENNE PEPPER

Cayenne pepper can be taken either as a drink or applied onto the skin as an ointment, depending on what condition you want to treat. But in the case of a cold we are going to take it as a drink.

Cayenne pepper can be bought in two different forms, either as a powder or a capsule. It is very much dependent on personal preference as to which form you buy. Both have there merits.

Myself, I prefer to take cayenne pepper in the powdered form. This is simply because I find it easier, if needed, to adjust the amount of cayenne I use.

And I also find the powder absorbs into the blood stream quicker which means it takes less time to feel its benefits.

So for this reason the following methods use powdered cayenne.

How to use cayenne pepper in a drink

The thing to bear in mind here is that cayenne pepper is very hot, and if you take too much in one go it can actually make you vomit. So the sensible thing is to start slowly with small amounts to allow your body to get used to it.

The preparation for the drink is very simple.

Add the cayenne pepper powder to a cup or glass, pour the required amount of liquid over the cayenne then let it rest for a minute. Stir the mixture well so that as much of the cayenne is absorbed into the liquid and then drink.

You may find it best to either continue stirring, or swirling, the mixture as you drink it to ensure the cayenne doesn't sink to the bottom of the cup.

Listed next are the various recipes for using cayenne pepper to treat a sore throat, the cold itself and then the cough that follows it.

CAYENNE FOR A SORE THROAT

When you feel the first signs of a sore throat the best thing to do is attack it straight away with dose of cayenne pepper.

The reason for this is that the primary compound of cayenne pepper is capsaicin which has both anti-bacterial and anti-fungal properties to it. Capsaicin stimulates the mucous membranes and reduces the sensation of pain from the inflammation caused by the soar throat.

Cayenne Pepper Tea

Ingredients:

1 cup of boiling water - let it cool a little first

½ teaspoon cayenne pepper powder

½ lemon (juice)

1 teaspoon of honey

Dash of salt

Firstly put the cayenne pepper powder into a cup, boil a kettle, let it cool down a little, then pour the water into a cup. Then add the juice from the lemon and the honey and stir till they are all mixed together.

As you drink the mixture keep stirring so that the cayenne doesn't sink to the bottom of the cup. Repeat this three times a day for maximum benefit and relieve the symptoms of the sore throat.

If you find ½ teaspoon of cayenne is too powerful for you at first, reduce the amount a little till you can tolerate it. Be aware though, if you make the mixture too weak you will not get the full benefit from it.

The cayenne pepper tea is actually the best method for relieving a sore throat instantly.

But, if you still cannot bear to drink it even after reducing the amount of cayenne pepper used then try making a gargle solution instead.

Cayenne Pepper Gargling Solution

Ingredients:

1 cup of boiling water - let it cool a little first

½ teaspoon cayenne pepper powder

½ lemon (juice)

Dash of salt

Mix all the ingredients together as above and then gargle with this solution every thirty minutes.

CAYENNE FOR A COLD

E ven as child I can remember being told to take plenty of Vitamin C whenever I was suffering from a cold or the flu.

What I have learned since is that if you add cayenne pepper to the Vitamin C you end up with a mixture that is so powerful it can actually stop a cold or flu in its tracks.

Why is this mixture so powerful?

Vitamin C is good at treating a cold because it is an antioxidant. But it is difficult for the body to retain Vitamin C in any large quantities.

Cayenne pepper, which is an accentuator medicinal spice, actually amplifies the nutritional qualities of whatever nutrient it is added to.

So the cayenne pepper amplifies the powerful

healing effects that are already there in Vitamin C, by allowing the body to absorb more of it, making it a very powerful combination for curing a cold or flu.

Here is how you make it:

Cayenne for Cold Relief

Ingredients

½ teaspoon cayenne pepper powder

3-4 oz of orange juice

You can use lemon juice, grapefruit juice or any other drink packed with Vitamin C, if you prefer. Stir the mixture together and then simply drink.

Most people find that the mixture of cayenne pepper powder with orange juice is far easier and nicer to drink than the cayenne and warm water mix.

CAYENNE FOR A COUGH

The end of a cold is normally followed by an irritating cough. This can be either a dry ticklish cough or a full chesty variety, but either way, it can be extremely irritating.

Just when your body needs rest to aid your recovery you are kept awake all night by a persistent cough.

There are some very good over the counter cough mixtures to be found, but they are mostly either expensive or make you drowsy and unable to drive or operate machinery.

But as we have already learned, cayenne pepper's warming effect has a powerful action on the mucous membrane which helps relieve your chest of congestion and phlegm, helping to put an end to your irritating cough.

So with that in mind I have given you two cayenne pepper recipes that will help ease or reduce the cough altogether.

Cayenne Cough Drink

Ingredients

¼ teaspoon cayenne pepper powder

2 tablespoons of warm to hot water

Add the ingredients to a cup or glass and stir well so that cayenne pepper is dissolved as much as possible.

Swallow the contents in in one gulp.

Repeat this procedure three times a day until the cough no longer persists.

Another very good recipe for relieving an irritating cough and getting a good nights sleep is the cayenne cough syrup.

Cayenne Cough Syrup

Ingredients

¼ teaspoon cayenne pepper powder

¼ teaspoon ground ginger

1 tablespoon honey

1 tablespoon apple cider vinegar

2 tablespoons water

Mix all the ingredients together, then take a teaspoon of the mixture three times a day.

Please remember, this is a medicine that will do you the world of good, and keep reminding yourself of that fact. Because, it has to be said, it is something of an acquired taste.

Please also bear in mind the cayenne pepper recipes shown here are only for a cough following a bad cold.

If you have had a cough that has lasted longer than a week or more and did not follow on from a cold you are advised to consult your doctor regarding this.

FREQUENTLY
ASKED QUESTIONS

Which is best, the capsule or powder?

That is really down to your own preference, but in my opinion I prefer cayenne pepper as a powder.

This is simply because I use different amount to treat different symptoms and I find the powder absorbs into my blood stream quicker.

How often should I take cayenne pepper?

This really depends on what symptoms you are taking cayenne pepper for. With regards to cold symptoms see the recipes in this book. If you just want to take cayenne pepper for its health benefits then one cup of cayenne pepper tea each day would be fine.

When should I take cayenne pepper?

You can take cayenne pepper anytime of the day that suits you. There are, however, times when it is advisable not to take cayenne pepper. I would avoid taking after a heavy meal, and certainly neither before or after any strenuous exercise.

How hot should the drink be?

Once again this depends on what you are taking cayenne pepper for. But generally speaking if you are taking the powder with water then the heat of the water is best somewhere between lukewarm and boiling.

Is cayenne powder from a supermarket okay?

Yes it is, but you won´t get the best result from using this variety. The reason for this is because it will more than likely have been irradiated. This is basically done to give it a longer shelf life, but in doing so it loses some of its potency.

The supermarket variety of cayenne powder is more suitable to be used as a spice to add flavor to food such as curries. That is not to say that you won´t get any benefit from this but it will be limited.

Where is the best place to buy cayenne powder?

The best place to buy cayenne powder would be from your local health food shop, or from an herbal wholesalers on-line website. You can even buy cayenne pepper powder from Amazon.com.

Which is the best cayenne powder to buy?

Cayenne is actually ranked by measuring the levels of capsaicin it contains. There are two methods of measuring these levels, the Gillette Method and the Scoville Heat Units (SHU). The Scoville measuring scale has become the most popular method.

Cayenne is rated from 30,000 to 50,000 SHUs. That is the rate I would recommend starting with, and all the recipes in this book use this rate.

If you look in your local health food shop, or online, you will find cayenne that is hotter than this. In fact it can go right up to 140,000 SHUs which, as you can imagine, is extremely hot. But, I would not recommend buying cayenne rated any higher than 50,000SHUs until you are completely comfortable with that level of heat. The old saying "buyer beware" is very apt with this situation.

Will cayenne pepper make me feel ill?

Taking cayenne pepper powder as a drink will certainly make your lips, mouth and tongue feel warm or a very slight burning sensation.

If you drink cayenne after any strenuous exercise you might well end up with a bad stomach ache.

But, if you take a large amount in one go it could make you vomit! Read the instructions in this book about starting small and building up the amount of cayenne you take.

OTHER HEALTH BENEFITS
OF CAYENNE PEPPER

As you read through this list of benefits you will begin to see why it was no exaggeration when I called cayenne pepper a miracle cure.

Heart and Cardiovascular

Cayenne is able to equalize the body's blood pressure by regulating the flow of blood from the head to the feet. This has an obviously beneficial effect on not only the heart itself, but also to the arteries, capillaries and nerves too.

Cholesterol can be lowered with regular use of cayenne pepper, it is also beneficial for all forms of heart disease, as well as preventing and treating blood clots.

It has been claimed that cayenne pepper can even stop an heart attack in its tracks.

Digestive System

Cayenne is very good at promoting digestion by stimulating the flow of saliva and enabling a feeble stomach to digest food more easily. It is also very good for the treatment of heartburn, dyspepsia and flatulence due to its carminative effect.

It can also aid the digestive system by rebuilding the tissues in the stomach to help heal the stomach and stomach ulcers.

Because cayenne pepper produces a natural feeling of warmth in your body this stimulates the motion of the intestines to help with the assimilation and elimination.

When used in larger quantities (above 20g) cayenne can be used as a laxative to induce frequent bowel movements. Cayenne can also be used for relieving sea-sickness too.

Immune System

Cayenne can help improve the whole immune system by alleviating allergies and muscle cramps and helping wounds to heal more quickly and without as much scarring.

It can also help ease the pain of rheumatism and arthritis, joint pains and swellings, as well chronic lumbago too.

Cayenne is good at helping to improve the health of the body's vital organs such as the kidney, spleen and pancreas. It can also be used to stimulate the gall bladder reflex.

When taken internally it is particularly good at treating the symptoms of colds as its warming effect has a powerful action on the mucous membrane.

Cancers

An article in the journal Cancer Research, reports on a study carried out by Dr Soren Lehmann of the Cedars-Sinai Medical Center in Los Angeles where he claims that the main ingredient in cayenne, capsaicin, was able to destroy cancer cells in the prostate.

He said, "Capsaicin led 80 percent of human prostate cancer cells, growing in mice, to commit suicide in a process known as apoptosis."

The study revealed that prostate cancer tumors in mice fed on capsaicin were about one-fifth the size of tumors in untreated mice.

BENEFITS AT A GLANCE

Stops heart attack instantly

Lowers blood pressure

Lowers cholesterol

Re-builds blood cells

Clears out arteries

Removes toxins from blood stream

Kills prostate cancer cells

Helps recovery from frostbite

Heals Hemorrhoids

Re-builds stomach tissue

Heals stomach ulcers

Improves circulation

Improves digestion

Relieves heartburn and indigestion

Soothes toothache

Relieves fever

Relieves a sore throat

Helps to ease and reduce a cough

Eases osteoarthritis and rheumatoid pain

Helps relieve shingles

Eases joint pains

Used as a laxative

Used to stop diarrhea

Heals cuts and wounds

Helps relieve malaria

SIDE EFFECTS AND WARNINGS

The main thing to stress here is that cayenne pepper, like anything beneficial, needs to be taken in moderation. It is also wise to start with a smaller dose and gradually build up to the required amount to avoid any discomfort.

Cayenne pepper is often taken as a powder, a pill or even whole. It can also be used as an ointment directly onto the skin.

When you first start taking cayenne pepper as a drink in its powdered form you will notice a warming or mild burning of the lips, mouth and throat. This is normal and should last for only a couple of minutes at the most.

Skin and eye irritation

After using powdered cayenne make sure to wash

your hands thoroughly as any contact to the eyes can cause very bad irritation. Be careful using it on your skin as an ointment as those with sensitive skin may find it can burn or itch.

Allergic Reaction

Before taking cayenne pepper it is best to check that you are not likely to suffer from an allergic reaction to it. Those people who are already allergic to chestnuts, latex, kiwis, avocados or bananas are more likely to be allergic to cayenne too.

The symptoms of cayenne allergy may include difficulty breathing, swelling of the throat, vomiting, hives and loss of consciousness. If you begin to suffer any of these symptoms after taking cayenne seek medical help urgently.

Gastrointestinal upset

Although cayenne pepper is in most cases a benefit to the digestive system for some people it may cause a mild irritation of the stomach.

This is often because too big a dose was taken in one go.

The way around this is to start with a small amount and slowly build up the dosage until you arrive at the desired amount.

It is also wise not to take cayenne pepper straight after doing any strenuous form of exercise as this will also cause you to suffer from stomach ache.

Other issues

It is not advisable to administer cayenne to children under the age of two.

If you are breastfeeding do not take cayenne orally.

If you are pregnant do not take cayenne without first consulting with your doctor.

Do not take large doses for any long periods of time as this can cause damage to your liver and kidneys.

Stop using at least two weeks before any surgery as cayenne can cause increased bleeding.

If you are taking any prescribed medication consult your doctor before using cayenne pepper as the capsicum in this herb can clash with other drugs.

DRUG COMPANIES

Having just read all about the amazing health qualities of cayenne peppers you are probably wondering why this knowledge isn't more widely known.

The truth is it's because the big drug companies don't want you to know. They make a lot of money from manufacturing and selling medicines because there is a lot of money to be made from health products. Or, to put it more accurately from products for ill-health.

So, you can see, it is not in their interest for you to know about other, often much cheaper, methods and products to relieve your illness.

And to some point that is quite understandable. The pharmaceutical industry employs huge numbers of highly trained scientists and technical staff to run their business. Their research and development budgets are massive and obviously all those costs have to be passed onto someone. Normally the end user – which is you!

So it is only natural that having made such a huge up-front investment they don't want people to know of other methods of finding a cure to their illness.

The other point to bear in mind here too, is that the pharmaceutical industry is actually a chemical industry. The end result is a drug, or chemical, that you ingest in your body.

And as we all know these drugs or chemicals can, and do, have their side effects.

For example. A couple of years back I came across a copy of the US edition of the Reader Digest, rather than the UK edition (now no longer published) that I was used to reading.

There was just something about this edition that seemed odd to me, although I couldn't put my finger on it at first.

It wasn't until flipping through the pages a good few times that I realized what the difference was.

Throughout the UK edition there would be pages of articles and stories separated by the odd page or two of adverts.

But in the US edition it was slightly different. It

also had all the pages of articles and stories, just like the UK edition, but when it featured an advert for a medical product, like lets say indigestion tablets, there followed two or three full pages of disclaimers.

The disclaimers were in such small type I had to strain my eyes to simply read them.

As America has more of a claims culture than the UK these pages were there to warn the consumer all about the different side effects of this particular product.

Page after page!

In the case of the indigestion tablets it even warned you that you could suffer with – wait for it – indigestion.

So what is the point of buying a product that the makers know, along with all its other side effects, could give you the very thing you are taking it to try and cure.

Absolute madness!

And yet it is these sort of products the majority of us turn to each and every time we want to relieve the symptom of our particular ailment.

Surely it is much better, for your body as well as your health, to use a natural product rather than a more chemical based one?

CONCLUSION

Thank you for buying and reading Cure Sore Throats, Colds and Coughs with Cayenne Pepper.

I am sure you will find the information contained within this book to be fascinating, and that you will look at the fiery hot cayenne pepper in a completely different light from now on.

I can honestly say that if you follow the advice and directions given within these pages you will quickly discover why I am so enthusiastic about using cayenne pepper.

I can personally testify to the benefits of cayenne pepper at curing the symptoms of a cold as I have not only benefited from it myself but also witnessed its amazing power with family members too.

If you have enjoyed reading this book and found the information helpful I would be grateful if you would add a review of it so other people might benefit from it also.

Thank you,

Nigel Thomas

ALSO BY THIS AUTHOR

The books listed below can be found at Amazon in their Kindle section.

How to Lower High Blood Pressure
using Cayenne Pepper

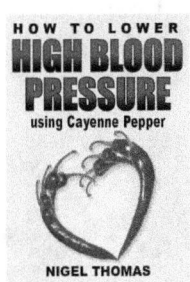

High blood pressure has become known as, "the silent killer," for a very good reason.

It is estimated that around one third of all adults suffer from high blood pressure.

Even more concerning is the fact that a great deal of them will be unaware they even suffer from the condition.

More people suffer from high blood pressure now than at any other time!

In this book you will learn:

What the effects of high blood pressure are.

How cayenne pepper is a natural cure for high blood pressure.

How to use cayenne pepper to lower high blood pressure

And, how to prevent getting high blood pressure

This is a GREAT little guide book for learning How to Lower High Blood Pressure Using Cayenne Pepper.

Affirmations for Health, Wealth and Happiness

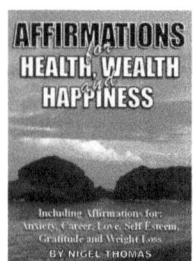

We are all looking for health, wealth and happiness - but few of us ever find it. Probably because we don´t know how to go about finding it.

But this illustrated book of affirmations will teach you how!

I am sure you have all heard of affirmations before, maybe even used one or two over the years, but did you ever realize how important affirmations are and the effect they have on you?

In this book you will learn:

Why affirmations are so important.

What positive affirmations are.

Why you should use them.

How often to use them . . .

. . . and, find examples of affirmations you can use for health, wealth and happiness, plus also affirmations for anxiety, career, love, self-esteem, gratitude and weight loss.

This is a GREAT little guide book of affirmations.